CLINICAL
EXAMINATION
SKILLS
FOR THE MRCP PACES EXAM

Dr. Deepa Iyer
MB BS, MRCP(UK)

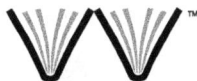

Whiteley Publishing

Published by Whiteley Publishing Ltd
First soft cover edition 2012

ISBN 978-1-908586-48-3
Deepa Iyer has asserted her right under the Copyright, Designs and Patents
Act 1988, to be identified as the author of this work.

Dedicated to my parents,
Dr. K Mohan Iyer
My biggest inspiration
and
Mrs. Nalini K Mohan
My biggest moral support

Dr. Kanishka Banerjee
My loving and caring husband
and
Mr. Rohit Iyer
My ever supportive brother

And to all my teachers who believed in me and taught me the value of
perseverance and integrity

Contents

Foreword

It is a very great pleasure to provide a foreword for this small but essential book. The author has produced a condensed blend of the best guidance from various sources and has created an excellent guide for the candidate preparing for clinical examinations. The style is clear, straightforward and practical. The content is traditional and conventional yet contemporary and resonant with modern bedside teaching in the UK. Dr Iyer's passion for the subject and insight into the needs of the candidates is apparent and adds a strong thread of relevance and authenticity to the content.

Though aimed primarily at candidates for the Royal Colleges of Physicians MRCP PACES exam the book has a generic function that is suitable for a wide range of clinical exams, including final undergraduate assessments, and is also a good aid memoire for established doctors who need to brush up their clinical technique. The author takes the reader through the five PACES stations, which provide the structure for the book. As well as direct advice on the technical aspects of the stations there are appropriate and subtle suggestions regarding conduct and approach that will be valuable to all readers, and particularly those who have trained in health systems outside the UK. The sections dealing with stations 2 and 4 will be especially valuable in that respect.

There is a plethora of publications that help candidates prepare for written higher examinations in Medicine but few that deal well with modern clinical examinations. This book meets that need and fills the gap in current provision for aspiring physicians working toward their formal qualifications.

Stephen Allen BSc MD FRCP MBA
Consultant Physician and Visiting Professor
The Royal Bournemouth Hospital

Preface

It is with great pleasure that I have compiled this humble book to help candidates giving the MRCP PACES exam. This book intends to take candidates back to the basics required to succeed at this particular hurdle.

The PACES exam is the only clinical part of the Diploma. It consists of 5 stations and each station is scored on 7 different skills. It is essential to achieve the minimum standard for each of the standard skills and also attain the minimum total score across the whole assessment to pass this exam.

This book takes candidates through all the clinical stations and goes through the examination sequence in detail. It is very important to be aware of the tiny details of clinical examination as these really count in this exam.

The examination techniques are described in great detail and include appropriate communication skills, to impress the importance of being courteous to your patients and not causing them any discomfort.

Practice is the main key to success and hence I would sincerely encourage everyone to get in touch with their local PACES teams and practice the art of examination and presentation.

I hope this book finds favour with everyone who reads it. I wish all the very best to everyone taking this exam.

Dr. Deepa Iyer

Acknowledgements

I am extremely grateful to everyone involved in making this book a reality. I send my undying gratitude to my parents, my husband and brother for all their support and guidance.

Also I extend my sincere thanks to all of my consultants for the long hours that they spent teaching me before my own exam, giving me invaluable advice and guidance. I have incorporated their invaluable words in this book and hope that they will be as useful to many candidates in the future as they were to me.

My gratitude would not be complete without thanking the innumerable patients we examined, particularly in view of the odd hours that we approached them to request for their help and for their patience with all of us.

Overview of the Exam

The MRCP PACES exam has been conducted since the early 2000's. It is very important for all candidates to be familiar with the structure of the exam. The exam consists of 5 stations of which stations 1 and 3 are the clinical examination stations, while station 2 and 4 are history taking and communication skills stations respectively. Station 5 amalgamates all skills involved in the above stations.

Station 1
- Respiratory system examination - 10 minutes
- Abdominal system examination - 10 minutes

Station 2
- History taking skills - 20 minutes

Station 3
- Cardiovascular system examination - 10 minutes
- Nervous system examination - 10 minutes

Station 4
- Communication skills and ethics - 20 minutes

Station 5
- Integrated clinical assessment
- *Brief clinical consultation 1 - 10 minutes*
- *Brief clinical consultation 2 - 10 minutes*

All candidates rotate through these stations and are given 5 minutes in between stations to make notes if necessary. This time also helps the candidate to collect their thoughts and to prepare for the next station.

Time is of the essence in this exam and so practice is essential. You should always aim to finish clinical examinations in the required time, so that you will be able to formulate a provisional or differential diagnosis.

Station 1
Abdominal and Respiratory System Examination

Abdominal Examination:

Introduction:

It is always important to greet the patient courteously. Ensure that the patient is lying flat on the bed, provided that they are able to lie flat and that the appropriate area is uncovered.

It is important to ask the men to take their shirts off and for women to be exposed adequately, whilst not compromising their dignity in any way. Always cover the patient when not examining the exposed area.

Introduce yourself to the patient and ensure that they understand what you are about to do before you launch into any examination.

Before touching the patient, make sure to use the hand gel by the end or side of the bed and warm your hands, especially if your hands are cold. Always ask the patient if he/she has pain or tenderness anywhere before you start the examination.

Examination:

1. Introduce yourself to the patient. Always be formal: *"I am Dr. ---------"*.

2. Let them know what you are about to do: *"I have been asked to examine your tummy. Would that be OK?"* This achieves verbal consent and initiates good communication.

3. Ask the patient if they are comfortable lying flat and ensure that the bed is adjusted if not already done. Remember to lay the patient flat for abdominal examination, unless told otherwise by the examiners or unless the patient expresses any distress or discomfort at being laid down.

4. Ask the patient if they have any pain or discomfort anywhere. Reassure them that you will try not to cause any discomfort and, should you do so, to let you know immediately.

5. Once you have established a rapport with your patient, expose the required area and tell the patient that you would like to stand at the end of the bed and start by simple observation.

6. Look around the bed and cabinet for any clues, such as: insulin pumps/injections, medicines, build up drinks, walking aids, blood glucose measuring devices, etc.

7. From the end of the bed ask the patient to take deep breaths and observe the abdomen to check if all segments are moving equally and symmetrically with respiration. Also ensure you check for the signs of recent weight loss with evidence of aproning of the skin on the abdomen.

8. Next ask the patient to cough to check for any hernias or any obvious abdominal masses which might become prominent.

9. Once you are happy with the observation, move closer to the patient, standing on their right side. At this point you can cover them up since you will be starting your examination with their hands.

10. *Start with the hands:*
-   Palms: erythema, Dupuytren's contractures, pallor, scars from previous surgery.
-   Nails: leuconychia, koilonychia, cyanosis, clubbing, paronychia, splinter haemorrhages.
-   Joints: Inflammation, swelling, deformities.
-   Skin: Dry, coarse skin, tightness, sclerodactyly, ulcers, infarcts, evidence of Raynaud's syndrome, colour changes, bruising, excoriation, pigmentation.
-   Ask the patient to hold their hands out and cock their wrists back to check for the hepatic flap or fine tremor.
-   Feel for the pulse and count for 10 seconds.
-   Examine the elbows and forearms for any arteriovenous fistulae, skin tightness, skin changes, needle marks and tattoos.

11. *Examining the face:*
- Eyes: evidence of icterus, pallor, xanthelasma.
- Nose: beaking, telangiectasia.
- Mouth: pallor, telangiectasia, cyanosis, gum hypertrophy, parotid enlargement.
- General skin appearance: tightness, pallor, icterus, spider naevi, cushingoid facies.

12. *Neck:*
- *Lymph nodes:* cervical chain, occipital nodes, supraclavicular fossae (remember Virchow's node).
- Evidence of previous central line scars, spider naevi, viral warts.

13. *Chest:*
- Gynaecomastia.
- Sparse body hair, loss of axillary hair.
- Spider naevi, excoriation, skin pigmentation, viral warts.
- Scars from previous tunnel line insertions, or presence of tunnel lines.

14. *Abdomen:*

Inspection:
- Movement with respiration.
- Evidence of fullness in any of the segments.
- Venous distension, caput medusa.
- Evidence of scars, previous surgery, peritoneal dialysis, ascitic drain sites, stoma sites, renal transplant scars and fullness, liver transplant scars, nephrectomy scars.

Palpation:
- Ensure your hands are warm before touching the patient.
- Superficial palpation: all 9 segments - right and left hypochondrium, right and left flank, right and left iliac fossa, the umbilical area, hypochondrium and the supra-pubic region.
- Deep palpation: all 9 segments.
- Palpation for the liver: from the right iliac fossa upwards to the right costal margin
- Ensure you comment on size, shape, consistency - firm/hard/ knobbly, pulsatile, tenderness.
- If enlarged, remember to count how many finger breadths from the right costal margin.

- Palpation for the spleen: from the right iliac fossa towards the left hypochondrium
- Ensure you comment on the above mentioned points for the spleen as well.
- Remember to turn the patient slightly to the right and palpate the left hypochondrium again – feel for the notch.
- Palpation for the kidneys: check for ballotability, palpable kidneys.
- Palpate under scars to check for masses.
- Establish movement with respiration, size and nature of palpable mass.

15. *Percussion:*
- Percuss for liver and splenic dullness.
- Percuss the midline to establish ascitic dullness and check for shifting dullness.
- It is not necessary to check for fluid thrill if you have established ascitic dullness.

16. *Auscultation:*
- Bowel sounds.
- Hepatic bruit.

Always thank the patient once you have finished the examination.

» *Presentation to the examiner:*

Everyone has their own method of presentation but the 2 most commonly used techniques are:

1. To start with the diagnosis and give your evidence for the same
2. To present in a systematic order and conclude with the diagnosis

To conclude your presentation, always tell the examiner what you would do to complete your clinical examination. For example:

"I would like to complete the examination by examining for generalised lymphadenopathy, examining the hernial orifices and doing a per rectal examination".

You will need to change your completion plan based on the case that you have examined. You may want to do a urine dipstick in some patients or examine other systems.

Flow Chart for Abdominal Examination

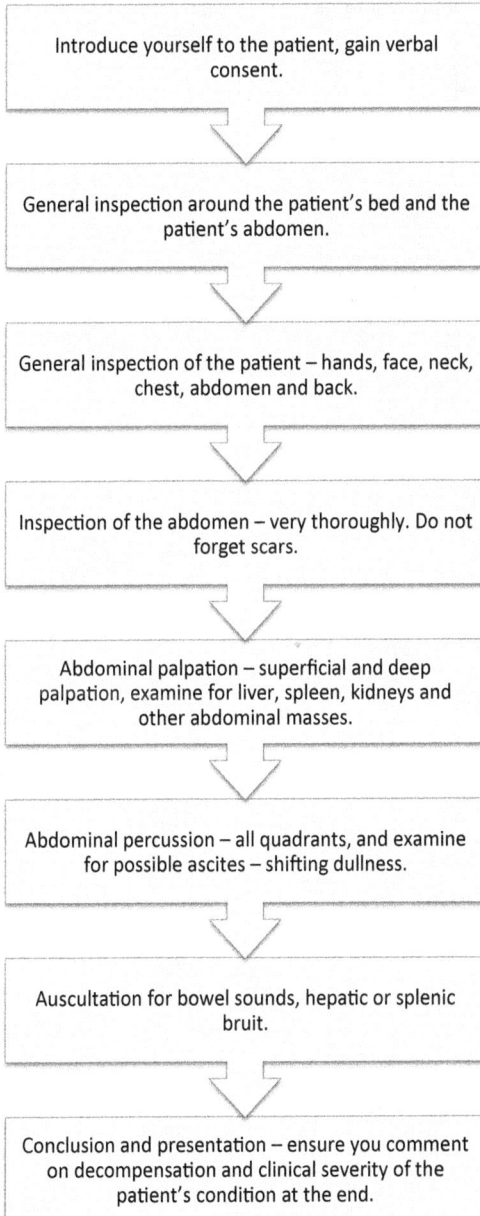

Introduce yourself to the patient, gain verbal consent.

⬇

General inspection around the patient's bed and the patient's abdomen.

⬇

General inspection of the patient – hands, face, neck, chest, abdomen and back.

⬇

Inspection of the abdomen – very thoroughly. Do not forget scars.

⬇

Abdominal palpation – superficial and deep palpation, examine for liver, spleen, kidneys and other abdominal masses.

⬇

Abdominal percussion – all quadrants, and examine for possible ascites – shifting dullness.

⬇

Auscultation for bowel sounds, hepatic or splenic bruit.

⬇

Conclusion and presentation – ensure you comment on decompensation and clinical severity of the patient's condition at the end.

Common Abdominal Cases:

1. Chronic liver disease - compensated or decompensated.
2. Hepatomegaly.
3. Splenomegaly.
4. Hepatosplenomegaly.
5. Polycystic kidney disease.
6. Organ transplants – liver/ kidney.
7. Haemochromotosis.
8. Primary biliary cirrhosis.
9. Inflammatory bowel disease.
10. Nephrotic syndrome.

Respiratory System Examination:

Introduction:

It is always important to greet the patient courteously. Ensure that the patient is comfortable sitting on the bed and is adequately exposed.

It is important to ask the men to take their shirts off and for women to be exposed adequately, whilst not compromising their dignity in any way. Always cover the patient when not examining the exposed area.

Introduce yourself to the patient and ensure that they understand what you are about to do before you launch into any examination.

Before touching the patient, make sure to use the hand gel by the end or side of the bed and warm your hands, especially if your hands are cold. Always ask the patient if he/she has pain or tenderness anywhere before you start the examination.

Examination:

1.   Introduce yourself to the patient. Always be formal: "*I am Dr. ------ ---*".

2.   Let them know what you are about to do: "*I have been asked to examine your chest. Would that be OK ?*" This achieves verbal consent and initiates good communication.

3.   Ask the patient if they are comfortable sitting on the bed and ensure that the bed is adjusted appropriately if this has not already been done.

4.   Ask the patient if they have any pain or discomfort anywhere. Reassure them that you will try not to cause any discomfort and, should you do so, to let you know immediately.

5.   Once you have established a rapport with your patient, expose the required area and tell the patient that you would like to stand at the end of the bed and start by simple observation.

6. Look around the bed for any clues, such as: inhalers, spacer devices, oxygen therapy, sputum pots, insulin pumps/ injections, medicines, build up drinks, walking aids, blood glucose measuring devices, etc.

7. From the end of the bed ask the patient to take deep breaths to check for symmetrical and equal respiration. Count the respiratory rate for 10 seconds.

8. Ask the patient to cough. This manoeuvre should reveal if they have bronchiectasis.

9. Once you are happy with the observation, move closer to the patient, standing on their right side. You can cover them up since you will be starting the next part of your examination with their hands.

10. *Start with the hands:*
-   *Palms*: capillary refill time, cyanosis, erythema, pallor.
-   *Nails*: cyanosis, clubbing, splinter haemorrhages, nicotine staining.
-   *Joints*: inflammation, swelling, deformities.
-   *Skin*: dry, coarse skin, tightness, sclerodactyly, ulcers, infarcts, rashes, evidence of Raynaud's syndrome, colour changes, bruising, excoriation, pigmentation.
-   Ask the patient to hold their hands out and cock their wrists back to check for the carbon dioxide retention flap or fine tremor secondary to salbutamol usage.
-   Feel for the pulse and count for 10 seconds.

11. *Examining the face:*
-   *Eyes*: evidence of icterus, pallor, xanthelasma, Horner's syndrome.
-   *Nose*: beaking, telangiectasia.
-   *Mouth*: pallor, telangiectasia, cyanosis, gum hypertrophy, thrush.
-   *General skin appearance*: tightness, pallor, icterus, spider naevi, cushingoid facies, cachexia, thinning of skin and bruising to indicate long term steroid usage.

12. *Neck:*
-   Lymph nodes – cervical chain, occipital nodes, supraclavicular fossae.
-   Evidence of previous central line scars, previous tracheotomy or tracheostomy scars, phrenic nerve crush.

- Tracheal position, tracheal tug.
- Jugular venous pressure

13. *Chest:*

Inspection:
- You can either start with anterior or posterior examination of the chest.
- Observe carefully for asymmetric chest expansion.
- Look very closely for scars – thoracoplasty, lobectomy, previous chest drains/ aspirations.
- Check the skin for telangiectasia, pigmentation, etc.

Palpation:
- Chest expansion: check in at least 3 areas, with equal distance from thumbs to midline.
- Tactile vocal fremitus.
- Apex beat, right ventricular heave.

Percussion:
- Percuss all segments of the lungs, comparing the right to the left.

Auscultation:
- Listen to all areas comparing the right to the left.
- Ask the patient to cough to check if crackles clear on coughing.
- Vocal resonance: *"Could you please say "99" every time you feel my stethoscope touch you?"*

Complete the examination by repeating this same sequence for the front or back of the chest, depending on what was first examined.

- Check for bipedal oedema

Always thank the patient once you have finished the examination.

» *Presentation to the examiner:*

To conclude your presentation, always tell the examiner what you would do to complete your clinical examination. For example:

> *"I would like to complete the examination by examining the sputum pot, looking at the patients observation chart – oxygen saturation, temperature and PEFR."*

Also explain if the patient has any evidence of right heart involvement or is compromised due to his/her respiratory condition.

Flow Chart for Respiratory Examination

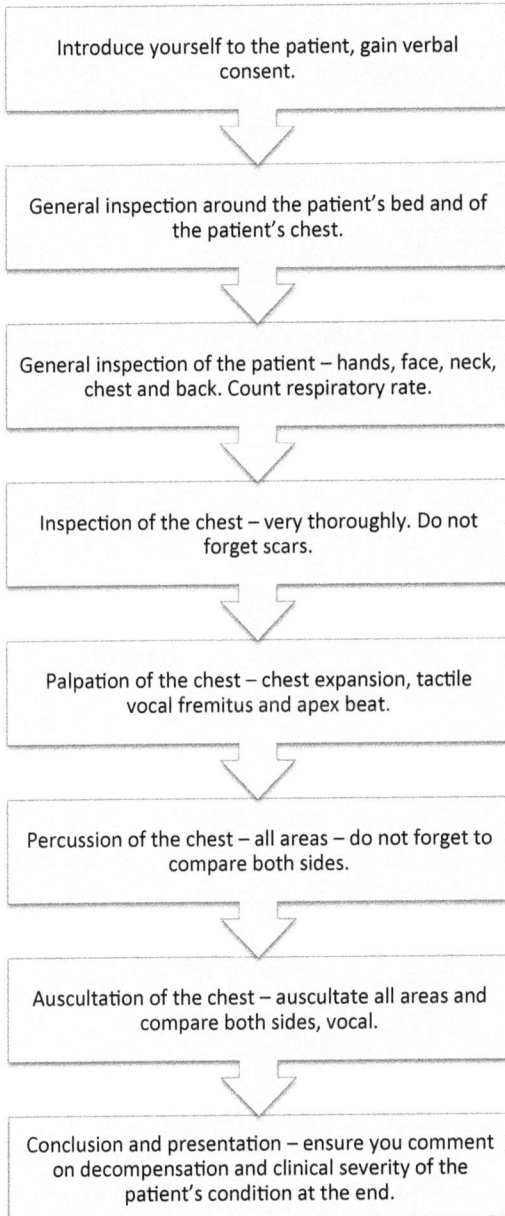

Introduce yourself to the patient, gain verbal consent.

Ⓥ

General inspection around the patient's bed and of the patient's chest.

Ⓥ

General inspection of the patient – hands, face, neck, chest and back. Count respiratory rate.

Ⓥ

Inspection of the chest – very thoroughly. Do not forget scars.

Ⓥ

Palpation of the chest – chest expansion, tactile vocal fremitus and apex beat.

Ⓥ

Percussion of the chest – all areas – do not forget to compare both sides.

Ⓥ

Auscultation of the chest – auscultate all areas and compare both sides, vocal.

Ⓥ

Conclusion and presentation – ensure you comment on decompensation and clinical severity of the patient's condition at the end.

Common Respiratory Cases:

1. Pulmonary fibrosis /interstitial lung disease.
2. Bronchiectasis.
3. Pleural effusion.
4. Pneumonectomy/lobectomy /lung transplant.
5. Chronic obstructive airways disease.
6. Mitotic lung lesion.
7. Cystic fibrosis.
8. Old tuberculosis.
9. Rheumatoid lung.
10. Consolidation.

Station 2
History Taking

Introduction:

This is one the easiest stations to gain marks. All of us take clinical histories from patients on a daily basis and so we should all be well prepared for this station.

It is very important to use the 5 minutes prior to entering the station to list all the possible differentials for the presentation. You can either prepare methodically by going through the systems or you can consider the commonest causes first. For example - if the patient has presented with syncope, you could either list the cardiovascular, neurological, endocrinological, infectious and other causes, or alternatively, you could make a list of the commonest causes of this symptom for the patients age/ sex/ presentation.

Always stick to the history taking structure, to ensure you ask all the relevant questions and complete the station:

1. Start with the presenting complaint and go through it in great detail. Even if you have established the cause, make sure you go through at least 3 differential causes.

2. Move on to the past medical history, ensuring that you ask about previous hospital admissions and previous surgery, even if minor.

3. Take a thorough medication history, including any herbal remedies or Chinese medication. Ask about any allergies to any drugs. If the patient does give you a history of allergy, ascertain what type of allergy and the severity. Ask if they have had any formal testing for this response.

4. Always remember the family history to ensure you cover any possible genetic diseases or any illness that could run in the family. If necessary be prepared to draw the genetic tree.

5. Move on to social history. Ask where the patient lives, with whom they live, who is their next of kin and other family members, including the number of children.

    Ask if they are in a committed relationship and, if so, for how long. If necessary ask if they had any other partners and any necessary sexual history.

    You should ask what their job is and for how long they have been doing it. In addition you should check if they have worked in any other jobs, eg. exposure to asbestos or paint, etc.

    Ask the patient if they smoke, how many cigarettes they smoke (if cigarettes) and how many years they have smoked (to calculate the pack years), if they have ever tried to give up and, if they failed, why so.

    Take a detailed alcohol consumption history: what they drink, how much they drink and if they have ever had a drinking problem. Be prepared to go through the CAGE questionnaire if necessary:

a. *Have you ever tried to Cut down on drinking?*
b. *Have you ever been Annoyed with people asking you to cut down?*
c. *Have you ever felt Guilty about drinking too much?*
d. *Have you ever used alcohol as an Eye opener?*

    Also ask about using recreational drugs and, if the patient does admit to have used them in the past, ask them for how long they have been clear.

6. Ask about travel history, both recently and in the past.

7. Ask about functional history: how the patient is managing at home, any help required, any aids used, etc.

8. Do not forget a thorough systems review. Go through all the systems in detail: headaches, visual disturbances or hearing problems, problems with swallowing, chest pains, shortness of breath, nausea or vomiting, abdominal pains, bowel disturbances, problems with micturition, joint pains, fevers, rashes, problems with mobility, weakness or sensory disturbances, etc.

9. Summarise the history to the patient before giving them a provisional or even a differential diagnosis.

10. Tell the patient how you would like to investigate them and give them a follow up plan. If you are referring them to a specialist, explain the necessity and how you plan to go about it and whether urgent or routine.

11. Ensure the patient understands your reasoning and check their understanding.

12. Thank the patient to conclude the consultation.

Once you have completed the station, you are given 1 minute to collect your thoughts when it would be advisable to write down your differential diagnoses and prepare for the questions to follow.

Flow Chart for History Taking

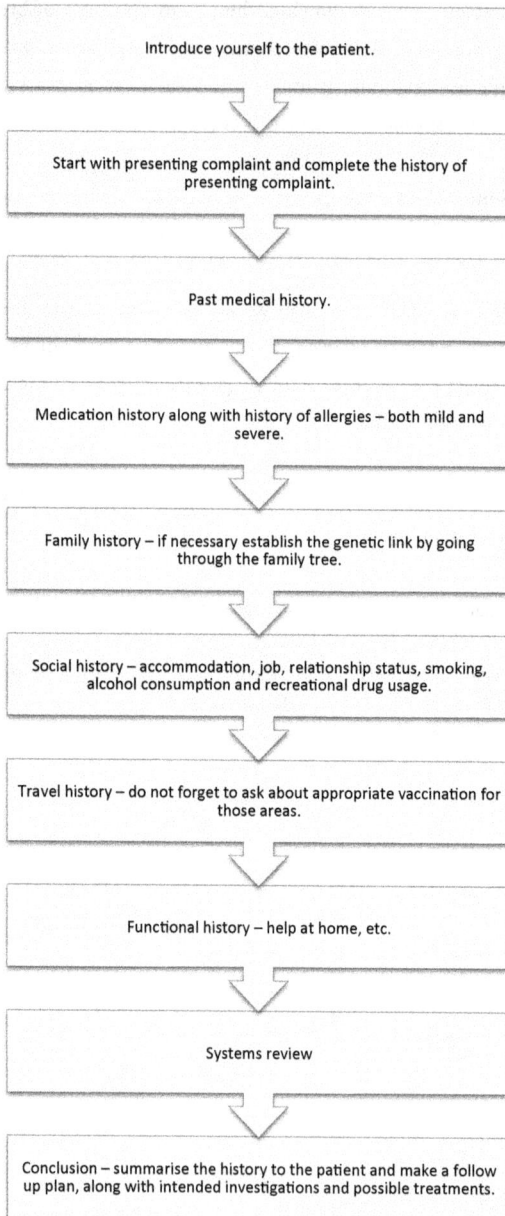

Introduce yourself to the patient.

⬇

Start with presenting complaint and complete the history of presenting complaint.

⬇

Past medical history.

⬇

Medication history along with history of allergies – both mild and severe.

⬇

Family history – if necessary establish the genetic link by going through the family tree.

⬇

Social history – accommodation, job, relationship status, smoking, alcohol consumption and recreational drug usage.

⬇

Travel history – do not forget to ask about appropriate vaccination for those areas.

⬇

Functional history – help at home, etc.

⬇

Systems review

⬇

Conclusion – summarise the history to the patient and make a follow up plan, along with intended investigations and possible treatments.

Station 3
Cardiovascular and Nervous System Examination

Cardiovascular System Examination:

Introduction:

It is always important to greet the patient courteously. Ensure that the patient is lying at 45 degrees on the bed and is adequately exposed.

It is important to ask the men to take their shirts off and for women to be exposed adequately, whilst not compromising their dignity in any way. Always cover the patient when not examining the exposed area.

Introduce yourself to the patient and ensure that they understand what you are about to do before you launch into any examination.

Before touching the patient, make sure to use the hand gel by the end or side of the bed and warm your hands, especially if your hands are cold. Always ask the patient if he/she has pain or tenderness anywhere before you start the examination.

Examination:

1. Introduce yourself to the patient. Always be formal: *"I am Dr. ---------"*.

2. Let the patient know what you are about to do: *"I have been asked to examine your heart – Would that be OK?"* This achieves verbal consent and initiates good communication.

3. Ask them if they are comfortable sitting at 45 degrees on the bed and, if so, ensure that the bed is adjusted appropriately if this has not already been done.

4. Ask the patient if they have any pain or discomfort anywhere. Reassure them that you will try not to cause any discomfort and, should you do so, to let you know immediately.

5. Once you have established a rapport with your patient, expose the required area and tell the patient that you would like to stand at the end of the bed and start by simple observation.

6. Look around the bed for any clues, such as: oxygen therapy, medications, GTN sprays, insulin pumps/injections, blood glucose measuring devices, etc. You can also note any obvious scars on the patient's chest and legs indicating a saphenous vein graft.

7. Once you are happy with the observation, move closer to the patient, standing on their right side. You can cover their exposed areas now as you will be starting your physical examination with their hands.

8. *Start with the hands:*
-   *Palms*: capillary refill time, cyanosis, pallor, Janeway lesions and Osler's nodes.
-   *Nails*: cyanosis, clubbing, splinter haemorrhages, nicotine staining.
-   *Joints*: inflammation, swelling, deformities.
-   *Skin*: dry, coarse skin, tightness, sclerodactyly, ulcers, infarcts, evidence of Raynaud's syndrome, colour changes, bruising, excoriation, pigmentation, tendon xanthomata.
-   Feel for the pulse and count for 10 seconds. Check for a collapsing pulse, after checking with the patient that they have no pain or discomfort in their shoulder. If they do have any discomfort, change sides or avoid doing it altogether.
-   Look for radial artery harvest scars or scars from previous angiography.

9. *Examining the face:*
-   *Eyes*: evidence of pallor, xanthelasma, corneal arcus.
-   *Nose*: beaking, telangiectasia.
-   *Mouth*: pallor, telangiectasia, cyanosis.
-   *General skin appearance*: tightness, pallor, cushingoid facies, cachexia, malar flush.

10. *Neck:*
-   Evidence of previous central line scars.
-   Jugular venous pressure
-   Carotid pulsations, especially if very prominent (Corrigan's sign).
-   Prominent jugular pulsations.

11. Cardiovascular system:

Inspection:

- Look very carefully for midline sternotomy scars, mitral valvotomy scars, etc.
- Look for visible pulsations: apical, carotid, etc.

Palpation:

- Feel for the apical impulse in the left fifth intercostal space just medial to the mid-clavicular line. Note if displaced. Turn the patient slightly to the left if necessary.
- Note the character of the impulse and check for apical–radial pulse mismatch.
- Check for heaves and thrills.

Auscultation:

- Always remember to feel the carotid pulse while auscultating the 4 areas of the heart.
- *Mitral area*: auscultate over the apex.
- Identify the first and second heart sounds and listen for murmurs.
- Change to the bell and ask the patient to turn slightly to the left and listen with the breath held in expiration for the mitral stenotic murmur.
- Always check for radiation of any murmurs.
- *Tricuspid area*: auscultate over the lower left sternal edge.
- Check for variation with respiration if a murmur is heard.
- *Pulmonary area*: auscultate over the left 2nd intercostal space.
- Check for variation of murmur with respiration.
- *Aortic area*: auscultate over the right 2nd intercostal space.
- Check for variation of murmur with respiration.
- Check for radiation to the carotids.
- When the patient sits up, ask them to bend forwards and hold their breath in expiration. Check for the regurgitant murmur of aortic incompetence. Remember to auscultate over the lower left sternal edge for the same.
- With the patient sitting forward, examine the lung bases for crackles and check for sacral oedema.
- Feel for bipedal oedema and for evidence of saphenous vein grafts.

Always thank the patient once you have finished the examination.

To conclude your presentation, always tell the examiner what you would do to complete your clinical examination. For example:

"I would like to complete the examination by looking at the observation chart for the temperature and blood pressure, would like to do a urine dipstick by the bed side to look for microscopic haematuria and perform a fundoscopy."

Also explain if the patient has any evidence of heart failure or any peripheral stigmata of infective endocarditis.

Flow Chart for Cardiovascular System Examination

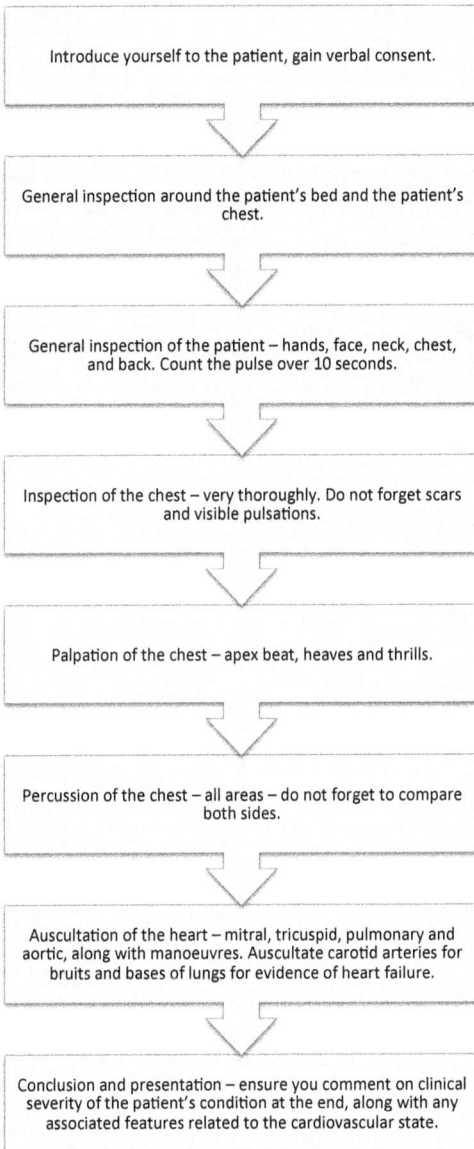

Introduce yourself to the patient, gain verbal consent.

↓

General inspection around the patient's bed and the patient's chest.

↓

General inspection of the patient – hands, face, neck, chest, and back. Count the pulse over 10 seconds.

↓

Inspection of the chest – very thoroughly. Do not forget scars and visible pulsations.

↓

Palpation of the chest – apex beat, heaves and thrills.

↓

Percussion of the chest – all areas – do not forget to compare both sides.

↓

Auscultation of the heart – mitral, tricuspid, pulmonary and aortic, along with manoeuvres. Auscultate carotid arteries for bruits and bases of lungs for evidence of heart failure.

↓

Conclusion and presentation – ensure you comment on clinical severity of the patient's condition at the end, along with any associated features related to the cardiovascular state.

Common Cardiovascular Cases:

1. Mitral regurgitation.
2. Mitral stenosis.
3. Aortic stenosis.
4. Aortic regurgitation.
5. Valve replacements – mitral or aortic.
6. Combined valve lesions.
7. Ventricular septal defect.
8. Fallot's tetralogy with Blalock Tausig's shunt.
9. Tricuspid/pulmonary regurgitation.
10. Rarer cases:
    -   Dextrocardia.
    -   Patent ductus arteriosis.
    -   Coarctation of aorta.
    -   Hypertrophic cardiomyopathy.

Central Nervous System Examination:

Introduction:

It is always important to greet the patient courteously. Ensure that the patient is comfortable sitting on the bed.

Introduce yourself to the patient and ensure that they understand what you are about to do before you launch into any examination.

Before touching the patient, make sure to use the hand gel by the end or side of the bed and warm your hands, especially if your hands are cold. Always ask the patient if he/she has pain or tenderness anywhere before you start the examination.

Examination:

1. Introduce yourself to the patient. Always be formal: "*I am Dr. --------*".

2. Let them know what you are about to do: "*I have been asked to examine the nerves of your face. Would that be OK?*" This achieves verbal consent and initiates good communication.

3. Ask the patient if they are comfortable sitting at the edge of the bed and adjust the bed appropriately if it has not already been done.

4. Ask the patient if they have any pain or discomfort anywhere. Reassure them that you will try not to cause any discomfort and, should you do so, to let you know immediately.

5. Once you have established a rapport with your patient, expose the required area and tell the patient that you would like to stand at the end of the bed and start by simple observation.

6. Look around the bed for any clues, such as: walking sticks (white indicating blindness/white with red band indicating blind and deaf), Braille books, insulin pumps/syringes, medications, etc.

7. Once you are happy with the observation, move closer to the patient and start the clinical examination:

Start with 3 questions:

a.   *"Did you have your breakfast this morning". If yes: "Could you smell your morning coffee OK? Have you noticed any change in the sense of your smell recently?"*

b.   *"Did you read the morning paper? Did you have any trouble with reading?"*

c.   *"Are you able to see my entire face? Is any part of my face missing?"*

Cranial Nerve Examination:

I:

- Smell: test the sensation of smell in each nostril.

II:

- Visual acuity: test vision in each eye separately. Tell the examiner that you would ideally assess the vision formally with a Snellen's chart.
- Visual fields: ensure you sit in front of the patient with just your knees touching the knees of the patient. Centre one of your fingers in between you and the patient and start wriggling it. Check the patient's field of vision against your own.
- Pupils: check light reflex, direct and consensual, size of pupils, differences in reaction, accommodation reflex.
- Fundoscopy: start with the red reflex and concentrate on the disc and retinal vessels.

III, IV,V:

- Eye positions: squints, ptosis, etc.
- Eye movements: check for diplopia, nystagmus, saccades, do the 'H' test. Do not forget to cover the eye to establish the side of the problem.

VI:

- Motor: ask the patient to clench teeth and then to open their jaw against resistance.
- Sensory: check all 3 divisions of the Trigeminal nerve – Ophthalmic, Maxillary and Mandibular. Tell the examiner that you would also check the corneal reflex.

VII:

- First observe for any obvious facial droop.
- Ask the patient to raise their eyebrows and wrinkle their forehead. Then ask them to puff their cheeks and blow and check that they are able to hold that position.

- Ask the patient to give you a broad smile and then show you their teeth. Remember in UMN (Upper Motor Neurone) lesions, the upper part of the face is spared.
- Tell the examiner that you would ideally test the taste sensation as well.

VIII:

- Check patient's hearing: rustle your fingers in each ear to begin and then close the opposite ear with a finger or palm to check hearing. Whisper a number in each ear with the opposite ear closed.
- Tell the examiner that you would ideally do the Rinne's and Weber's test to establish sensorineural or conductive deafness.

IX and X:

- Ask the patient to say 'Ah', to check palatal movement.
- Tell the examiner that you would ideally check the gag reflex.

XI:

- Ask the patient to shrug their shoulders.
- Ask the patient to move their head against resistance. Do not forget to feel for the opposite sternocleidomastoid muscle to ensure it is taut.

XII:

- Ask the patient to stick their tongue out and move it from side to side.
- Ask them to push against your finger with their tongue against their cheek.

Always thank the patient once you have finished the examination.

» Presentation to the examiner:

To conclude your presentation, always tell the examiner what you would do to complete your clinical examination. For example:

"I would like to complete the examination by examining the patient's arms and legs neurologically and examining other relevant systems."

Also comment if the patient is compensating by using aids.

Flow Chart for Cranial Nerve Examination

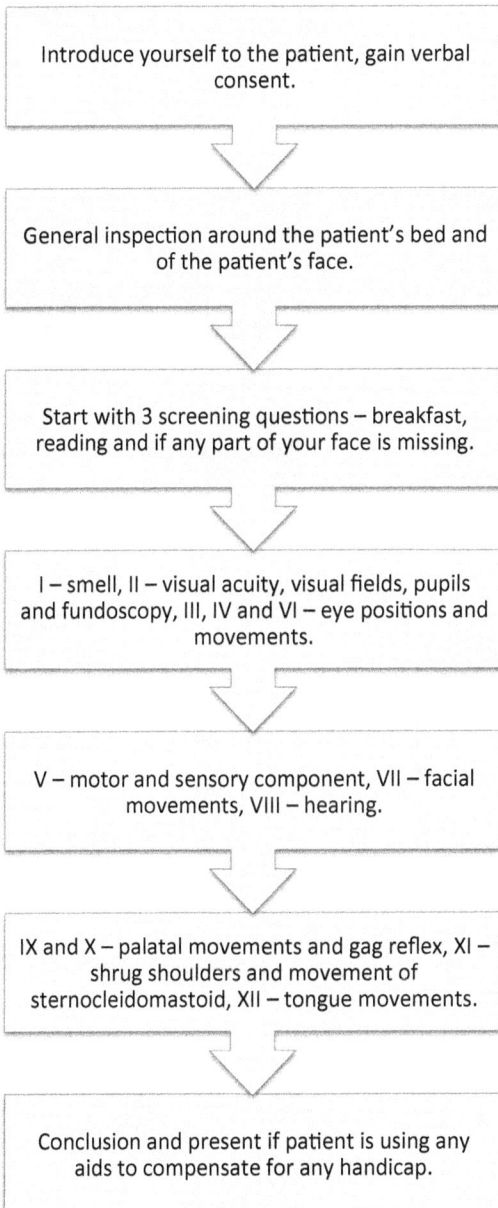

Introduce yourself to the patient, gain verbal consent.

⬇

General inspection around the patient's bed and of the patient's face.

⬇

Start with 3 screening questions – breakfast, reading and if any part of your face is missing.

⬇

I – smell, II – visual acuity, visual fields, pupils and fundoscopy, III, IV and VI – eye positions and movements.

⬇

V – motor and sensory component, VII – facial movements, VIII – hearing.

⬇

IX and X – palatal movements and gag reflex, XI – shrug shoulders and movement of sternocleidomastoid, XII – tongue movements.

⬇

Conclusion and present if patient is using any aids to compensate for any handicap.

Upper Limb Examination:

Introduction:

It is always important to greet the patient courteously. Ensure that the patient is comfortable on the bed and is adequately exposed.

It is important to ask the men to take their shirts off and for women to be exposed adequately, whilst not compromising their dignity in any way. Always cover the patient when not examining the exposed area.

Introduce yourself to the patient and ensure that they understand what you are about to do before you launch into any examination.

Before touching the patient, make sure to use the hand gel by the end or side of the bed and warm your hands, especially if your hands are cold. Always ask the patient if he/she has pain or tenderness anywhere before you start the examination.

Examination:

1.   Introduce yourself to the patient. Always be formal: "*I am Dr. --------*".

2.   Let them know what you are about to do: "*I have been asked to examine your arms. Would that be OK?*". This achieves verbal consent and initiates good communication.

3.   Ask the patient if they are comfortable on the bed and ensure that the bed is adjusted appropriately if this has not already been done.

4.   Ask the patient if they have any pain or discomfort anywhere. Reassure them that you will try not to cause any discomfort and, should you do so, to let you know immediately.

5.   Once you have established a rapport with your patient, expose the required area and tell the patient that you would like to stand at the end of the bed and start by simple observation.

6. Look around the bed for any clues, such as: walking sticks (white indicating blindness/white with red band indicating blind and deaf), Braille books, insulin pumps/syringes, medications, etc.

7. Once you are happy with the observation, move closer to the patient to start the physical examination:

Inspection:
- Observe closely for any fasciculations, muscle wasting, scars, postural deformities, aids etc.
- Check for pronator drift.

Tone:
- Ask the patient to relax and let their arms go floppy.
- Move the patient's arms gently to assess tone. Move one arm at a time.
- Grade it according to the MRC grading.
- Ensure that the patient does not experience any discomfort.

Power:
- Explain that you would like to test the patient's strength in different muscles.
- Start with the shoulders. Ask the patient to shrug their shoulders and to resist you pushing them up or down.
- Ask them to bend their arms at their elbows and then to pull your hands towards them and then to push you away. Remember to stabilise their elbow with your other hand – check each arm at a time.
- Ask the patient to make fists and cock their wrists upwards. Ask them to resist your force while you try to move their wrists up or down.
- Ask the patient to spread their fingers out wide and to resist your attempt to move them inwards.
- Ask the patient to spread their fingers out wide and resist your attempt to move them downwards at the metacarpophalangeal joints.
- Lastly, ask the patient to squeeze your fingers.

Reflexes:
- Explain to the patient what you are about to do: *"I would like to check your reflexes with this tendon hammer. It does not cause any pain or discomfort"*.

- *Biceps reflex*: remember to place your thumb on the biceps tendon and stroke your thumb with the tendon hammer.
- *Triceps reflex:* easier to check with patients arms crossed on their chest.
- *Supinator reflex:* remember to place your index finger on the supinator tendon and stroke your finger with the tendon hammer.

Co-ordination:
- Ask the patient to use the tip of their index finger and touch the tip of their nose and then to touch the tip of your index finger. Tell them to do this as fast as possible.
- Check for dysdiadochokinesis.

Sensation:
- Check the patient's sensation on forehead to compare to their upper limbs.
- *Fine touch*: use a cotton wool and check dermatomally for sensory loss.
- *Pin prick*: use a neurological pin to assess if the patient perceives it as sharp or dull.
- *Joint position sense*: start with the thumb and if absent, move to the wrist and so on and so forth.

Vibration sense:
- Start on the first metacarpophalangeal joint and move towards the wrist for the best bony prominence. Ask the patient to also confirm when they stop feeling the vibration.
- Check for patient's functional status – ability to do their buttons/ write/ lift their cups, etc.
- Tell the examiner that you would ideally test for change in temperature perception.
- Always check for functional status in all neurological examinations: Writing, doing buttons and holding cups.

Always thank the patient once you have finished the examination.

To conclude your presentation, always tell the examiner what you would do to complete your clinical examination. For example:

"I would like to complete the examination by examining the patient's legs neurologically and examining other relevant systems."

Also comment if the patient is compensating by using aids.

Flow Chart for Upper Limb Examination

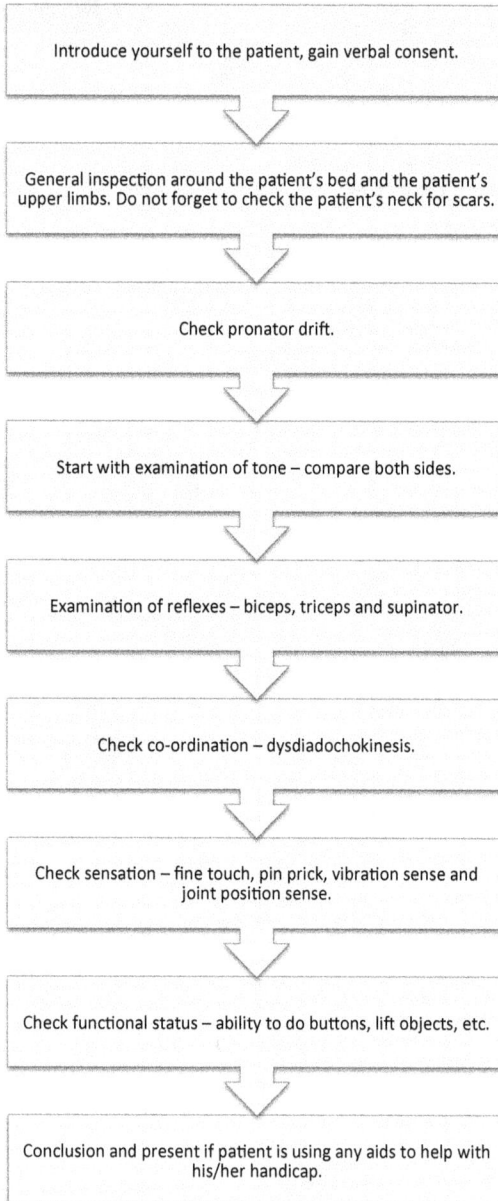

Introduce yourself to the patient, gain verbal consent.

General inspection around the patient's bed and the patient's upper limbs. Do not forget to check the patient's neck for scars.

Check pronator drift.

Start with examination of tone – compare both sides.

Examination of reflexes – biceps, triceps and supinator.

Check co-ordination – dysdiadochokinesis.

Check sensation – fine touch, pin prick, vibration sense and joint position sense.

Check functional status – ability to do buttons, lift objects, etc.

Conclusion and present if patient is using any aids to help with his/her handicap.

Lower Limb Examination:

Introduction:

It is always important to greet the patient courteously. Ensure that the patient is comfortable on the bed and is adequately exposed.

It is important to ask the patients to take their trousers off but leave their undergarments on, ensuring that you are not compromising their dignity in anyway. Always cover them up whilst not examining the exposed area.

Introduce yourself to the patient and ensure that they understand what you are about to do before you launch into any examination.

Before touching the patient, make sure to use the hand gel by the end or side of the bed and warm your hands, especially if your hands are cold. Always ask the patient if he/she has pain or tenderness anywhere before you start the examination.

Examination:

1. Introduce yourself to the patient. Always be formal: "*I am Dr. --------*".

2. Let the patient know what you are about to do: "*I have been asked to examine your legs. Would that be OK?*". This achieves verbal consent and initiates good communication.

3. Ask them if they are comfortable on the bed and ensure that the bed is adjusted appropriately if this has not already been done.

4. Ask the patient if they have any pain or discomfort anywhere. Reassure them that you will try not to cause any discomfort and, should you do so, to let you know immediately.

5. Once you have established a rapport with your patient, expose the required area and tell the patient that you would like to stand at the end of the bed and start by simple observation.

6. Look around the bed for any clues, such as: walking sticks (white indicating blindness/ white with red band indicating blind and deaf), Braille books, insulin pumps/syringes, medications, etc.

7. Once you are happy with the observation, move closer to the patient to start the physical examination:

Inspection:
- Observe closely for any fasciculations, muscle wasting, scars, postural deformities, aids etc.
- Ask the patient to stand up first and ensure they are steady on their feet.
- Get them to stand with their feet close together.
- Ask them to extend their arms and then to close their eyes to check for Romberg's sign.
- If they are steady, then proceed to ask them to take a few steps to examine their gait.
- Ask them to turn around gently and then to walk as if they were walking on a tight rope to check tandem gait.

While the patient is standing, examine their back to look for scars or any obvious deformities.

Ask the patient to sit on the bed with their legs rested on the bed.

Tone:
- Ask the patient to relax and let their legs go floppy.
- Ensure they are not in any pain or discomfort and move their legs gently to check the tone.
- Place your hand on the patient's knee and move the knee gently from side to side.
- Place your hand behind the patient's knee and raise it quickly to look for any evidence of spasticity.
- Grade tone according to the MRC grading.
- Check for ankle clonus at this stage.

Power:
- Tell the patient that you wish to test the strength in their legs.
- Ask them to raise their leg away upwards without bending their knee and to keep it there.
- Ask them to resist your force to push them upwards or downwards.

- Then ask them to bend their knees and, whilst stabilising the knee joint, ask them to pull your hand towards their buttock and then to push away. Repeat on the other side.
- Ask the patient to straighten their legs and move their foot toward their face and resist your hand.
- Then ask them to push on your hands like a pedal.
- Finally ask the patient to move only their big toe towards their face and to resist your finger.

Reflexes:
- *Knee jerk:* bend the patient's knee and support it with your hand from behind the knee.
- *Ankle jerk:* bend the patients knee and ask them to let it flop outwards. This could be awkward if not well practiced.
- *Plantar reflex:* use the orange stick to check this.

Co-ordination:
- Ask the patient to do the heel – shin test.

Sensation:
- Check the patient's sensation on forehead to compare to their lower limbs.
- *Fine touch:* use cotton wool and check dermatomally for sensory loss.
- *Pin prick:* use a neurological pin to assess if the patient perceives it as sharp or dull.
- *Joint position sense:* start with the big toe and if absent move to the ankle and so on and so forth.
- *Vibration sense:* start on the first metatarsophalangeal joint and move towards the malleoli for the best bony prominence. Ask the patient to also confirm when they stop feeling the vibration.

Tell the examiner that you would ideally test for change in temperature perception.

Always thank the patient once you have finished the examination.

» *Presentation to the examiner:*

To conclude your presentation, always tell the examiner what you would do to complete your clinical examination. For example:

"I would like to complete the examination by examining the patient's arms neurologically and examining other relevant systems."

Also comment if the patient is compensating by using aids.

Flow Chart for Lower Limb Examination

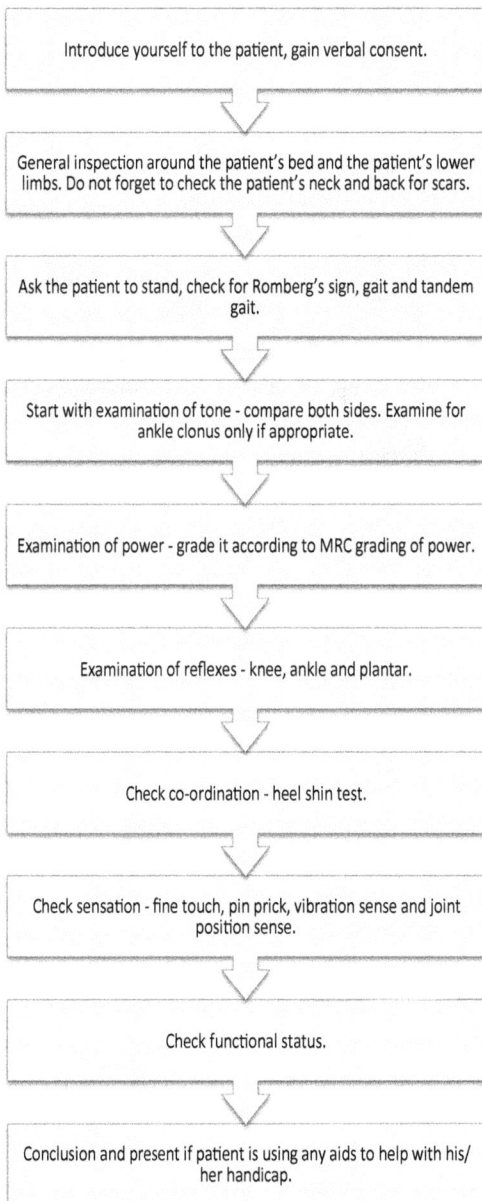

Introduce yourself to the patient, gain verbal consent.

General inspection around the patient's bed and the patient's lower limbs. Do not forget to check the patient's neck and back for scars.

Ask the patient to stand, check for Romberg's sign, gait and tandem gait.

Start with examination of tone - compare both sides. Examine for ankle clonus only if appropriate.

Examination of power - grade it according to MRC grading of power.

Examination of reflexes - knee, ankle and plantar.

Check co-ordination - heel shin test.

Check sensation - fine touch, pin prick, vibration sense and joint position sense.

Check functional status.

Conclusion and present if patient is using any aids to help with his/her handicap.

Common Nervous System Cases:

1. Cerebellar syndrome.
2. Peripheral neuropathy – motor/ sensory/sensorimotor.
3. Hemiplegia.
4. Charcot-Marie-Tooth disease.
5. Parkinson's disease.
6. Myotonic dystrophy.
7. Visual field defect/ocular palsy.
8. Spastic paraparesis.
9. Facial nerve palsy.
10. Other cases:
   - Motor neurone disease.
   - Mononeuropathies – ulnar nerve palsy/radial nerve palsy/ common peroneal nerve palsy/carpal tunnel syndrome.
   - Friedrich's ataxia.
   - Horner's syndrome.
   - Polio.
   - Cervical myelopathy.
   - Cerebellopontine angle lesion.
   - Absent ankle jerks with extensor plantars.
   - Cranial nerve lesions.

Station 4
Communication Skills

Introduction:

Familiarise yourself with the ethics and the law in the country of examination. It is essential that you remember the 4 pillars of medical ethics:

1. *Autonomy:* always respect the patient's decisions, even if they appear unreasonable, provided that the patient is competent.

2. *Beneficence:* always consider the patient's best interests first.

3. *Non maleficence:* never do wrong or harm to the patient.

4. *Justice:* ensure that resources are used justly and think about the well being of the whole population.

Examination:

1. Start by introducing yourself formally: *"Good morning/afternoon Mr/ Mrs..., my name is Dr..., I am the senior house officer/ Registrar in this clinic and I work with the consultant in charge of your care"*.
2. Remember empathy goes a long way in a breaking bad news scenario.
3. Ask if they are alone and if they need someone with them. Also enquire how they have travelled to your clinic, to ensure they are safe to drive back after receiving bad news.
4. Always check their knowledge of the situation and how much they are already aware of, before giving any information.
5. Ask of the patient's understanding of their problem if it is a case of breaking bad news or a long term illness.
6. Once you have gained an understanding of how much they patient is aware, you can then summarise what they already know and go on to explain investigations or talk about the problem you are meant to discuss.
7. Always ensure you are aware of the patient's ideas, concerns and expectations throughout the consultation.
8. Addressing patient's concerns is of top priority. Do not forget to check with the patient regularly, to make sure that they are following all you are saying.

9. In the case of an angry patient, allow them to talk and express their frustration. Never interrupt a patient who is giving you information.
10. Always encourage patients to ask as many questions as they wish.
11. When the 2 minute bell goes, always ask the patient for their concerns and address them. If you have not been able to complete your explanation, make a follow up plan, offer leaflets and websites that might be useful to them. In addition, remember there are always specialist nurses that you can refer the patients to.
12. Try hard to be reassuring, but do not be overly reassuring which could be misconstrued as false hope. Always be honest and truthful and remember that sometimes facts have to be stated as they are to get the necessary impact.
13. Thank the patient once you complete the station.

You will have 1 minute to collect your thoughts before the examiners ask questions.

Station 5
Brief Clinical Consultations

Brief Clinical Consultations:
(Rheumatology / Dermatology / Endocrinology / Ophthalmology / General Medicine)

Introduction:

It is important to remember that the majority of the marks in this exam are earned in this station. It is the most difficult station in the exam, as it requires assessment of all the skills to be available and to be used appropriately. Candidates are expected to take a brief history, do a specific examination and advise the patient on a suitable management plan, all within 8 minutes.

It is essential to remain calm and use the 5 minutes before entering the station to formulate a thorough plan and have a set of differential diagnoses in mind. The cases are normally straightforward but it is very important to have alternative possible diagnoses ready to discuss.

Remember that time is of the essence in this station, so once you establish the presenting complaint, request permission from the patient to start examination whilst continuing to ask questions. It would be worthwhile practising timing in this station. Limit the first 2 minutes to establishing the presenting complaint. Try to go through the entire history in order whilst examining the patient.

When the 2 minute reminder is given, ensure that you ask the patient for his/ her concerns and address their concerns immediately. The failure to do this is one of the most common errors which can be avoided easily.

Examination:

1. You would have already introduced yourself to the patient and established a rapport while trying to listen to the presenting complaint.

2. Always tell the patient clearly what you would like to examine and expose appropriately.

3. Formulate a general plan of examination for station 5.

Rheumatology:

1. *Start with the hands:*

- *Palms*: erythema, Dupuytren's contractures, pallor, vasculitic lesions, scars from carpal tunnel surgery.
- *Nails*: koilonychia, cyanosis, clubbing, paronychia, pitting, onycholysis, hyperkeratosis, periungual fibromas.
- *Fingers*: Bouchard's nodes, Heberden's nodes.
- *Joints*: inflammation, swelling, deformities (swan neck), Boutonniere's, Z thumbs, wrist subluxation, ulnar deviation at wrist and MCP's with volar subluxation.
- *Skin*: dry, coarse skin, tightness, sclerodactyly, ulcers, infarcts, evidence of Raynaud's syndrome, colour changes, bruising, excoriation, pigmentation.
- Feel for the pulse and count for 10 seconds.
- Examine the elbows and forearms for any rheumatoid nodules, skin and joint laxity, skin tightness, psoriatic patches, skin changes.
- Also assess function in hands if there is evidence of arthritis: power grip, precision grip, doing buttons, using a key, picking up coins.
- Assess sensation if necessary.
- Assess Tinel's, Froment's and Phalen's test if necessary.

2. *Examination of the face and neck:*

- *Eyes*: evidence of pallor, xanthelasma, corneal arcus, evidence of keratoconjunctivitis, dry eyes.
- *Nose*: beaking, telangiectasia, deformity.
- *Mouth*: pallor, telangiectasia, cyanosis.
- *General skin appearance*: tightness, pallor, cushingoid facies, cachexia, thinning of skin, bruising, skin laxity, yellow discoloration, dry skin, eczema etc.

3. *Examination of the rest of the body:*

- Examine each joint individually to assess its involvement and disease state. Look for signs of inflammation, tenderness and temperature.
- Establish which type of arthritis or rheumatological problem the patient has.
- Remember it could be a case of mixed connective tissue disease, so could have features of many conditions.

- Do not forget to assess functional state.
- It is also important to comment on disease activity and complications secondary to treatment for eg. skin thinning and bruising due to steroids.
- Look for scars of tendon transfers/carpal tunnel release/joint replacements.
- Ensure you are well versed with the systemic manifestations of the different rheumatological conditions. If you do not get the time to examine it, do tell the patient that you would have done so, had you had the time.
- Do not forget to look for signs of lupus, including discoid lupus. It is important to be aware of the multisystem involvement with lupus and read up about the criteria for its diagnosis.

Common Rheumatological Cases:

1. Rheumatoid arthritis.
2. Psoriatic arthropathy.
3. Polymyositis/dermatomyositis.
4. Systemic lupus erthyematosus/discoid lupus.
5. Systemic sclerosis/CREST syndrome.
6. Gout.
7. Ankylosing spondylitis.
8. Osteoarthritis.
9. Proximal myopathy.
10. Other cases:
    - Charcot's joint.
    - Paget's disease.
    - Vasculitis.
    - Jaccoud's arthropathy.
    - Marfan's syndrome.
    - Mixed connective tissue disease.

Dermatology:

Start with the hands:

- *Palms:* erythema, pallor.
- *Nails:* koilonychia, cyanosis, clubbing, paronychia, pitting, onycholysis, hyperkeratosis.
- *Fingers:* Bouchard's nodes, Heberden's nodes.
- *Joints:* inflammation, swelling, deformities (swan neck), Boutonniere's, Z thumbs, wrist subluxation, ulnar deviation at wrist and MCP's with volar subluxation.
- *Skin:* dry, coarse skin, tightness, sclerodactyly, ulcers, infarcts, evidence of Raynaud's syndrome, colour changes, bruising, excoriation, pigmentation.
- Feel for the pulse and count for 10 seconds.
- Examine the elbows and forearms for any rheumatoid nodules, skin and joint laxity, skin tightness, psoriatic patches, skin changes.
- Also assess function in hands if there is evidence of arthritis: power grip, precision grip, doing buttons, using a key, picking up coins.
- Assess sensation if necessary.

Examination of the face and neck:

- *Eyes:* evidence of pallor, xanthelasma, corneal arcus, evidence of keratoconjunctivitis, dry eyes, iritis.
- *Nose:* beaking, telangiectasia, deformity.
- *Mouth:* pallor, telangiectasia, cyanosis.
- *General skin appearance:* tightness, pallor, cushingoid facies, cachexia, thinning of skin, bruising, etc.

Examine the skin for evidence of psoriasis and establish what type it is:

- Look for associated arthropathy and also look for complications.
- If the patient has evidence of psoriasis, do not forget to look for other sites of involvement like behind the ears, navel and scalp.
- Also look for Koebner's phenomenon.
- Remember to examine both hands and feet, including nails, in such patients.

Again remember to assess function and establish any multisystem involvement.

Common Dermatology Cases:

1. Psoriasis.
2. Eczema.
3. Dermatomyositis.
4. Tuberous sclerosis.
5. Systemic sclerosis/CREST Syndrome.
6. Neurofibromatosis.
7. Vitiligo.
8. Raynaud's phenomenon.
9. Henoch-Schonlein purpura.
10. Other cases:
    - Urticaria.
    - Osler-Weber-Rendu syndrome.
    - Gouty tophi.
    - Ehler-Danlos syndrome.
    - Pseudoxanthoma elasticum.
    - Diabetic dermopathy/necrobiosis lipoidica diabeticorum.
    - Skin malignancy: basal cell carcinoma/squamous cell carcinoma/malignant melanoma.

Endocrinology:

1. *Start with the hands:*

   - *Palms:* erythema, pallor, fine tremor, sweaty palms, doughy hands, ill fitting rings – tight rings indicating enlargement of hands.
   - *Nails:* koilonychia, cyanosis, clubbing.
   - *Fingers:* Bouchard's nodes, Heberden's nodes, finger pricks from testing for diabetes.
   - *Joints:* inflammation, swelling, deformities (swan neck), Boutonniere's, Z thumbs, wrist subluxation, ulnar deviation at wrist and MCP's with volar subluxation.
   - *Skin:* dry, coarse skin, tightness, sclerodactyly, ulcers, infarcts, evidence of Raynaud's syndrome, colour changes, bruising, excoriation, pigmentation.
   - Feel for the pulse and count for 10 seconds. Establish if the patient is in atrial fibrillation.
   - Examine the elbows and forearms for any rheumatoid nodules, skin and joint laxity, skin tightness, psoriatic patches, skin changes.
   - Assess sensation if necessary.

2. *Examination of the face and neck:*

   - *Eyes:* evidence of pallor, xanthelasma, corneal arcus, eye movements, diplopia, lid lag, proptosis, exophthalmos.
   - *Nose:* beaking, telangiectasia, deformity.
   - *Mouth:* pallor, telangiectasia, cyanosis.
   - *General skin appearance:* tightness, pallor, cushingoid facies, cachexia, thinning of skin, bruising, fat pad, abdominal striae, muscle wasting, proximal myopathy.

3. *Ensure that you have practiced thoroughly for examination of the thyroid:*

   - Starting with inspection of any lump.
   - Ask the patient to swallow to check for movement of the lump on deglutition.
   - Then move behind the patient and warm your hands before palpating the thyroid.
   - Feel the isthmus, followed by the lobes and assess for lumps and tenderness.

- Repeat the swallow test.
- Palpate for lymph nodes.
- Percuss the midline for retrosternal extension and auscultate for bruits.
- Then look for pretibial myxoedema and examine reflexes.
- Remember to present your findings in a systematic fashion to ensure you have diagnosed the thyroid state of the patient – euthyroid/ hypothyroid/ hyperthyroid.

Common Endocrinological Cases:

1. Acromegaly.
2. Grave's disease/goitre/exophthalmos.
3. Hyperthyroidism/hypothyroidism.
4. Cushing's syndrome.
5. Addison's disease.
6. Klinefelter's syndrome.
7. Turner's syndrome.
8. Hypopituitarism.
9. Pseudohypoparathyroidism.
10. Others:
   - Diabetes.
   - Gynaecomastia.

Ophthalmology:

1. *General examination as before. You may need to do a fundoscopy to establish the problem:*

Ensure patient is seated comfortably on the chair.

- Explain the procedure to the patient: "*I need to examine the back of your eye. This would involve me shining this bright light into your eyes. This does no cause pain, but may be slightly uncomfortable. I will also require you to move your eyes during the procedure, but I will give you instructions as we go along. You can blink and breathe normally, but please do not move your head. I will be coming very close to you and the room will be darkened to allow me to ensure clear visibility of the back of your eye. If at any time, you wish me to stop, please let me know.*"
- Having explained the procedure, ensure the room is dark, with the lights turned off.
- Check that you have looked at the Ophthalmoscope and adjusted the settings to suit your vision.
- Start with the red reflex and then move closer to the patient.
- The examiners will let you know which pupil is dilated, so proceed to examine the dilated one.
- Aim the ophthalmoscope towards the opposite ear, which will help you focus on the disc. Trace the blood vessels from the disc and examine all four quadrants accordingly.

- Ask the patient to look to the left, to the right, to look up and down, to ensure all areas are thoroughly examined.
- Ask the patient to look directly at the light, to look for macular involvement.

2. Do not forget to formulate a management plan and address the patients concerns.

3. If unable to complete the examination, you can always address the patients concerns first and then say what you would ideally do to complete the examination.

Remember that the examiner has only 2 minutes to ask questions, so keep your answers to the point.

Common Ophthalmological Cases:

1. Diabetic retinopathy.
2. Hypertensive retinopathy.
3. Retinitis pigmentosa.
4. Optic atrophy
5. Myasthenia gravis.
6. Ocular palsy.
7. Old choroiditis.
8. Retinal artery/vein occlusion.
9. Visual field defect.
10. Others:
    - Cataracts.
    - Glaucoma.
    - Abnormal pupils – Holmes-Adie pupil, Horner's syndrome, Argyll-Robertson pupil, III Nerve palsy.
    - Age related macular degeneration.

Helpful tips:

1. Always be courteous to the patients and ensure good bedside manners.

2. Practice the art of presentation in front of the mirror and with colleagues.

3. Dress comfortably in formal clothing. For female candidates remember to dress bare below the elbows, wear no jewellery on your fingers and don't forget a watch for timing the pulse or respiratory rate.

4. Try to go on a PACES course. It will give you great insight into the exam and also give you a chance to see the different cases, including some rare ones.

5. It is impressive to remember the patient's name when presenting their case to an examiner.

6. Always time yourself while practising, as it is very important to try and finish the examination on time.

7. Be up to date with current guidelines for management of common problems including medical emergencies.

8. Make sure you are aware of the criteria for diagnosis of common conditions: Rheumatoid Arthritis/ SLE, etc.

9. While studying always make note of the 3 most common differentials for presentations. For example: the most common causes for Hepatomegaly include:
   - Cirrhosis of the liver.
   - Mitotic lesions in the liver.
   - Congestive cardiac failure.

10. Be familiar with common causes first before mentioning rarer causes for the cases.

11. Remember that you will be presenting the case in front of the patient so be cautious while describing your finding. For example, if the patient is obese and has Cushing's syndrome, do not present that this patient is "fat" or "obese". It would be more professional to say. "*This patient appears to have a raised body mass index*". Avoid any sort of derogatory terms during your presentation.

12. Do not make the mistake of taking too long to present your case, as the examiners have only 4 minutes in the clinical stations and 2 minutes in station 5 to question you. Give them the positive findings and the important negatives.

13. Never argue with the examiners even if you feel you were in the right. They are much more experienced than you and have been involved in medicine a lot longer than you have.

14. Always remain honest. It is very easy to be confidently wrong and that is a very easy trait for examiners to pick up on.

15. It helps to remain calm, though easier said than done. Try breathing exercises and try to have a good night's sleep prior to the exam.

16. The only way to ensure success in this exam is with practice. Form a group and encourage colleagues with positive criticism as this not only helps you get through this exam, it also makes you a better and more caring doctor.

17. This exam can be an enjoyable experience if approached with the right attitude. It ensures that candidates have the required skills to run a medical "take" not only with the right skills and knowledge but also with the right attitude to the patients.

Other reading:

1. Oxford Handbook of Clinical Medicine, 8th edition.

2. Cases for PACES, Stephen Hoole, Andrew Fry, Daniel Hodson and Rachel Davies

3. Kumar and Clark, Textbook of Clinical Medicine, 7th edition.

4. Clinical Medicine for the MRCP PACES Pack: 1-2 (Oxford Specialty Training: Revision Texts) by Gautam Mehta, Bilal Iqbal and Deborah Bowman

5. Aid to the MRCP Paces: Volume 1: Stations 1, 3 and 5 v. 1 by Bob Ryder, Afzal Mir and Anne Freeman

6. An Aid to the MRCP Paces: Volume 2: Stations 2 and 4 v. 2 by Dev Banerjee, Robert E. J. Ryder, M. Afzal Mir and E. Anne Freeman

7. MRCP Paces Ethics and Communication Skills (Master Pass) by Iqbal Khan

8. 250 Cases in Clinical Medicine (MRCP Study Guides) by Ragavendra R. Baliga